MINDFUL ANXIETY PANACEA

By
Roberta Kimberly

MINDFUL ANXIETY 1
WHAT IS ANXIETY? 1
Chapter Two 1
UNDERSTANDING YOUR ANXIETY 1
Chapter Three 1
Mindful Breathing Techniques 1
Chapter four 1
BENEFITS OF MAP 1
Chapter Five 1
TAKING THE STEP 1
Chapter One 1

Chapter One

MINDFUL ANXIETY

Mindful Anxiety Panacea (MAP) is a holistic approach to managing anxiety and stress. MAP is an evidence-based approach that combines mindfulness practices, cognitive-behavioral strategies, and positive lifestyle changes to reduce anxiety and improve overall mental health.

MAP teaches individuals to recognize, accept, and address the physical, mental, and emotional symptoms of anxiety.

This helps individuals to become aware of their thoughts, feelings, and body sensations in the present moment and to respond to them in helpful ways.

MAP also encourages individuals to pay attention to how their environment, lifestyle, relationships, and behavior contribute to their anxiety.

This helps them to identify and modify any unhealthy behaviors that may be contributing to their anxiety, such as unhealthy eating, lack of exercise, and social avoidance.

MAP also focuses on building resilience and

coping skills, such as problem-solving, self-care, relaxation, and positive self-talk.

By learning to use these skills, individuals can become more aware of and better equipped to manage their anxious feelings.

Overall, MAP is a holistic approach to managing anxiety that helps individuals to identify and address the causes of their anxiety, while also cultivating resilience and healthy coping strategies.

Once upon a time, there lived a young man named Ian who was constantly plagued by anxiety. He was so overwhelmed by his anxiety that he could not enjoy a single day without worrying about something.

One day, a wise old man approached Ian and told

him about a special remedy for his anxiety: Mindful Anxiety Panace.
 The old man said that if Ian were to take the remedy, he would find relief from his worries and be able to enjoy life to the fullest.
 Ian was skeptical at first, but the old man was so convincing that he decided to give it a try. He followed the old man's instructions and started practicing mindfulness every day.
He paid attention to his thoughts, feelings, and body sensations without judgment. He also practiced deep breathing and relaxation techniques. Soon, Ian noticed a difference. He felt calmer and more focused.
His worries and anxieties seemed to fade away. He was able to enjoy his days

and even look forward to
the future.
 He thanked the old man
for introducing him to
Mindful Anxiety Panace
and continued to practice
mindfulness every day.
Over time, he gained
more control over his
anxiety and was able to
live a happier, more
fulfilling life.
The moral of this story is
that as humans, it is
normal to be anxious
about things especially if
they are not going the way
we want them.
But we should never let
too much Anxiety into our
lives because we would
never appreciate and
enjoy the blessings we
have around us instead
our minds would be
focused on things we do
not have, or things that
are not working our ways
and that will steal away

the joy and happiness of
the present.
This story also teaches
solutions to Mindful
Anxiety. even if you are
suffering from Mindful
Anxiety, you can
overcome it by taking
some steps which will be
further explained as you
continue reading.

WHAT IS ANXIETY?

Anxiety is a normal
emotion characterized by
feelings of worry, fear, and
uneasiness. It is a natural
stress response and can
be beneficial, alerting us
to potential danger and
motivating us to take
action.
Still, when anxiety
becomes inordinate and
patient, it can intrude with
daily life and exercise.
Anxiety disorders are the

most common mental
health disorders and affect
millions of people
worldwide.
Common symptoms of
anxiety include excessive
worrying, restlessness,
difficulty concentrating,
and irritability.
Treatment for anxiety may
include psychotherapy,
medication, or a
combination of both.
Benefits of Mindfulness

Mindfulness is an ancient
practice that has been
around for centuries, and
its benefits are just
beginning to be
recognized by modern
science.
Mindfulness is the practice
of being aware and
present at the moment,
without judgment or
expectation.
 It involves paying
attention to one's

thoughts, feelings, and
sensations in the present
moment, without
comparing them to the
past or worrying about the
future.
Practicing mindfulness
has numerous benefits,
both physical and mental.
Physically, mindfulness
can help improve physical
health by reducing stress,
increasing relaxation, and
improving sleep.
 It can also help manage
chronic pain, improve the
immune system, and
reduce blood pressure.
Mentally, mindfulness can
help reduce anxiety and
depression, increase
focus and attention, and
improve overall emotional
well-being.
 It can also help with self-
acceptance and self-
compassion, and increase
overall psychological
resilience.

Mindfulness can also help improve relationships by enabling us to be more present and compassionate with ourselves and others. Overall, mindfulness can help us to live more fully in the present moment and to become more aware of our thoughts, feelings, and sensations.
It can help to create a sense of peace and well-being that can be applied to all aspects of life.

Chapter Two

UNDERSTANDING YOUR ANXIETY

Understanding your anxiety is key to managing and overcoming it.
The more you understand the nature of anxiety and

its causes, the better equipped you will be to recognize and address its symptoms. Anxiety is an emotion characterized by feelings of tension, worry, and unease.
It is a normal stress response, but when it becomes excessive and persistent, it can become a disorder.
Anxiety can manifest itself in physical, behavioral, and mental symptoms, such as difficulty sleeping, difficulty concentrating, fatigue, irritability, and restlessness.
Anxiety can be caused by a variety of factors, including genetics, environmental stressors, and life experiences.
It is important to identify and address the root cause of your anxiety to effectively manage it. For example, if you are feeling

anxious due to a traumatic event, talking to a therapist or joining a support group may be helpful.

It is also important to practice self-care, such as getting enough sleep, engaging in physical activity, and eating a healthy diet. Additionally, learning to manage stress and developing effective coping skills can help reduce anxiety.

Mindfulness and relaxation techniques, such as deep breathing and meditation, can also help manage anxiety. Lastly, it is important to remember that excess anxiety doesn't proffer solutions to problems but instead degenerates into bigger problems, it is best to kick it out as soon as we notice it setting in, you can do this by seeking help, never assume you can handle it alone, speak with experts, seek therapy.

Identifying Your Anxiety Triggers

Anxiety can be debilitating and can negatively affect your daily life. To overcome this, it's important to identify what triggers your anxiety. Identifying your anxiety triggers can help you to better manage and cope with your anxiety. One way to identify your anxiety triggers is to keep a journal. Write down when you are feeling anxious and what was going on at the time. Note any physical or emotional sensations that you experienced, such as a racing heart or thoughts of fear or dread. This will enable you to understand patterns in your anxiety. Another way to identify your anxiety triggers is to talk to a mental health professional.

 A therapist can help you to identify situations or events that may be triggering your anxiety. They can also help you to understand why you may be feeling anxious in certain situations. Lastly, it's important to practice self-care.

Make sure to get enough sleep and exercise, eat healthy foods, and find time to relax and do things that you enjoy. This can help to reduce stress and can prevent your anxiety from getting worse. Identifying your anxiety triggers can help you to manage your anxiety more effectively. It's important to remember that everyone experiences anxiety differently, and what works for Mr. A may not work for Mr. B so you need to identify what triggers your anxiety to know how best to deal with it.

Assessing Your Psychological State

Assessing your psychological state is an important part of maintaining mental health and well-being. Taking the time to check in with yourself regularly can help you identify any areas of concern and make proactive steps to address them. Here are some simple steps you can take to assess your psychological state:

1. Take an honest look at your thoughts. Are your thoughts mostly positive or negative? Do you find yourself frequently

ruminating on the same worries or anxieties? Are you having difficulty focusing on tasks?
 2. Check in with your emotions. Are you feeling overwhelmed or stressed out? Are you feeling optimistic? Are your emotions in balance, or do they seem to fluctuate?
3. Reflect on your behavior. Are you engaging in healthy activities and behaviors, such as exercise, eating nutritious foods, and getting enough rest? Are you avoiding activities that could be detrimental to your mental health, such as using drugs or alcohol?
4. Assess your relationships. Are you feeling connected and supported by your friends and family? Are there any areas of conflict or tension

that need to be
addressed?

5. Evaluate your overall
outlook. Are you feeling
confident in your abilities
and motivated to pursue
your set goals in life? Self-
evaluation will enable you
to discover on time if there
is any area of concern to
proffer lasting solutions or
get books like this to take
you through steps that will
help you out.

Chapter Three

Mindful Strategies

1. Make Time for
Meditation: Taking time
out of your day to
meditate can be a great
way to become more
mindful. Allocate a few
minutes each day to sit
and focus on your breath
and clear your mind.

2. Live in the Moment:
Take time to enjoy the
small moments in life and
pay attention to the
details. Focus on the
present moment instead
of worrying about the
future or ruminating over
the past.
3. Be Aware of Your
Thoughts: Instead of
letting your thoughts run
away with you, take a step
back and observe them.
Notice when you are
having unhelpful or
negative thoughts, and try
to challenge them.
4. Notice Your Emotions:
Pay attention to how you
are feeling and what
triggers those emotions.
Be aware of your
emotional reactions and
try to understand them.
5. Practice Gratitude:
Keeping a gratitude
journal can be a great way
to become more mindful.

Spend a few minutes each day writing down the things you are thankful for.
 6. Eat Mindfully: Instead of gobbling down your food, savor each bite and be aware of your hunger and fullness levels. Take time to enjoy the flavors and textures.
7. Take a Break: No matter how busy your daily schedule is always take time out to relax, excessive stress increases your chances of getting anxiety disorder.

Mindful Breathing Techniques

Mindful breathing is an essential practice for maintaining a healthy body and mind. It involves focusing on the breath and using it as a tool to bring awareness to the present moment.

1. Begin in a comfortable seated position. Close your eyes and focus on your breath.

2. Start by taking a few deep breaths. Feel the air coming in and out of your body.

3. Notice the sensations in your body as you inhale and exhale.

4. Position one of your hands on your chest and position the other on your tummy. Concentrate on the movement of your breath as your stomach and chest rise and fall.

5. If your mind starts to wander, simply bring your attention back to your breath.

6. Continue breathing deeply and slowly, focusing on the sensations of your inhalation and exhalation.

7. Take a few moments to simply observe your breath and be present at the moment. 8. When you're finished, slowly open your eyes and take a few moments to take in your surroundings.
Grounding Exercises

1. Take a few deep breaths. Close your eyes and focus on the breath, feel your body sink into the ground.
2. Take a few moments to identify different parts of your body that are touching the ground. Notice how it feels.
 3. Visualize roots growing from the soles of your feet, connecting to the Earth and anchoring you to the ground.
4. Place your hands on the ground and feel the energy of the Earth flowing through you.

5. Spend some time focusing on the sensation of being securely grounded.

6. As you feel more and more connected to the ground, take a few moments to think of all the wonderful things you're grateful for in your life.

7. When you're ready, slowly open your eyes and take a few more deep breaths.

Stress Reduction Exercise

Stress reduction exercises can help you manage stress in your life and improve your overall well-being.

Many different types of stress reduction exercises can be done, such as yoga, meditation, deep breathing, progressive muscle relaxation, and mindfulness.

Yoga is a great way to reduce stress and increase flexibility. It helps to improve balance, strength, and coordination and can provide an overall sense of well-being. During yoga, different poses are held for several minutes and can also help to reduce muscle tension. Meditation is a great way to relax and clear your mind. It can be done for just a few minutes or longer periods. During meditation, focus on your breathing and allow yourself to observe your thoughts without judgment or attachment.

Deep breathing is a simple but effective way to reduce stress. It involves taking slow, deep breaths that fill your abdomen and chest. Focus on the sensation of your breath and the feeling of your body as your chest rises and falls.

Progressive muscle relaxation is a type of relaxation technique that helps to reduce muscle tension. It involves tensing and relaxing different muscle groups, such as your arms, legs, and neck. This aids in the reduction of stress and maximizes rest.

Chapter four

BENEFITS OF MAP

The Mindful Anxiety Panacea is a powerful tool for reducing anxiety and helping individuals gain control over their emotions and reactions.

It provides a holistic approach to tackling anxiety, focusing on activities, techniques, and strategies that can help the individual become more aware of their thoughts and feelings and to gain control over them. The Mindful Anxiety Panacea is a great option for those looking for an alternative to traditional therapeutic approaches to managing anxiety. It is an effective and empowering approach that can help anyone to reduce their anxiety and improve their well-being.

Taking the next step can be intimidating, but it is essential to achieving your goals. Whether you are starting a new job, beginning a new relationship, or taking on a new project, it is important to be confident and prepared. The first step in taking the next step is to

assess your skills and abilities.
What do you need to learn or do differently to succeed? What resources do you have available to help you in this endeavor? Once you have identified the skills and resources you need, it is time to create a plan.
What are the things you must do to meet your target in life? Are there any obstacles that could prevent you from achieving them? Constructing a vivid plan and strategy that can help you remain motivated and focused.
 Finally, it is important to stay positive and believe in yourself. Even if something doesn't go as planned, don't give up.
A setback is not a sign of failure, but rather an opportunity to learn and

grow. Taking the next step can be a challenging process, but it is necessary for success. With the proper resources, a solid plan, and a positive attitude, you can make it happen.

Taking the next step on mindful anxiety panacea means becoming more aware of how your thoughts, emotions, and behavior influence your ability to cope with anxiety.

This could involve recognizing the triggers for your anxiety and working towards managing them more effectively. It could also involve learning more about mindfulness and using it to help manage and reduce your anxiety. Additionally, it could include making lifestyle changes that can reduce

stress and promote better
overall mental health,
such as getting more
sleep, exercising
regularly, eating a
balanced diet, and
reducing your caffeine and
alcohol intake.
Finally, it could mean
seeking out professional
help if needed, such as
consulting with a therapist
or counselor who
specializes in anxiety.
Taking the next step on
mindful anxiety panacea
can help you to better
understand and manage
your anxiety and gain
more control over your
life.

Chapter Five

TAKING THE STEP

Mindfulness is a powerful tool that can help move us forward in life. It can help us be more aware of our thoughts, feelings, and actions, so we can respond to life's challenges positively and healthily.
Here are some tips to help you move forward with mindfulness:
1. Take Time for Self-Care: Make sure to take time for yourself and do activities that make you feel relaxed, such as yoga, meditation, reading, or listening to music. Taking time for yourself can help you become more aware of your

thoughts and feelings, so you can mindfully respond to them.
2. Practice Acceptance: Accepting your thoughts and feelings without judgment can help you move forward with mindfulness.
Instead of worrying about the future, take the time to be present in the moment and observe your thoughts and feelings without judgment.
 3. Focus on the Positive: Instead of dwelling on the negative, focus on the positive aspects of life. This can help you stay grounded in the present moment and move forward with mindfulness.
 4. Take Breaks: Taking regular breaks throughout the day can help clear your mind and reset your focus. When you take a break, take a few

moments to be mindful
and
Mindfulness is an
important tool for
managing stress,
developing resilience, and
leading a healthier
lifestyle. Moving forward
with mindfulness involves
committing to practice
mindfulness regularly.
 This can be done through
meditation, yoga, mindful
eating, or other activities
that help to focus on the
present moment. Start by
setting realistic goals and
allowing yourself to be
kind to yourself.
Begin with a few minutes
a day and gradually
increase the time. There is
no need to pressure
yourself to achieve
perfection. As you
become more comfortable
with mindfulness, you can
incorporate it into your
daily routine.

Incorporate mindfulness into your life by focusing on your breathing, allowing yourself to be in the present moment, and taking time to appreciate the simple things in life. Find ways to practice gratitude and be kind to yourself.

When you find yourself overwhelmed or stressed, use mindfulness to help ground yourself. Quietly take a few breaths and focus on the present moment.

Remember that the current moment does not define you and that you are capable of handling the situation. Finally, take some time to reflect on your mindfulness practice each day.

Notice how it has helped you manage stress and become more resilient. Celebrate the small

successes and
acknowledge when you've
had a disappointment but
know it is not the end of
the road for you but only a
challenge that should be
overcome.
 You should Recognize
when you are stuck in a
negative thought pattern
and take a moment to
pause.
Honestly, ruminate on the
best things you should do
at the moment. Notice the
thoughts and feelings that
come up and make space
for them. Don't judge or
try to control them, just
observe and be curious.
Once you start to become
aware of your thoughts
and feelings, you can
begin to make changes.
Begin with setting realistic,
achievable goals you can
decide to start in a little bit
for yourself.

These could be anything
from getting up fifteen
minutes earlier each day
to eating more fruits and
vegetables.
 As you start to make
progress, you can
gradually increase the
difficulty of your goals.
Finally, practice self-
compassion. Be kind and
understanding to yourself.
Remind yourself that you
are doing the best you can
and that it is okay to make
mistakes. With self-
compassion,